Alvaro Carlos Galdos Riveros
Eliane Souza Moura
Evillin da Silva Lima

The role of pharmacotherapy in the treatment of metabolic syndrome

Alvaro Carlos Galdos Riveros
Eliane Souza Moura
Evillin da Silva Lima

The role of pharmacotherapy in the treatment of metabolic syndrome

Pharmacological aspects

ScienciaScripts

Imprint

Any brand names and product names mentioned in this book are subject to trademark, brand or patent protection and are trademarks or registered trademarks of their respective holders. The use of brand names, product names, common names, trade names, product descriptions etc. even without a particular marking in this work is in no way to be construed to mean that such names may be regarded as unrestricted in respect of trademark and brand protection legislation and could thus be used by anyone.

Cover image: www.ingimage.com

This book is a translation from the original published under ISBN 978-3-330-76517-7.

Publisher:
Sciencia Scripts
is a trademark of
Dodo Books Indian Ocean Ltd. and OmniScriptum S.R.L publishing group

120 High Road, East Finchley, London, N2 9ED, United Kingdom
Str. Armeneasca 28/1, office 1, Chisinau MD-2012, Republic of Moldova, Europe
Printed at: see last page
ISBN: 978-620-8-10323-1

First to God, who gave us strength in the most difficult moments of our lives. To our family and to everyone who directly or indirectly contributed to this work.'

ACKNOWLEDGMENTS

First of all, we would like to thank God, who allowed us to dream and make our dream come true. To our parents, who accompanied us on this journey, supporting us and for all their dedication. To our family for their understanding in times of absence and for their constant support and affection.

"Don't confuse defeat with failure or victory with success. In the life of a champion there will always be some defeats, just as in the life of a loser there will always be victories. The difference is that, while champions grow in defeats, losers settle in victories. "

(Roberto Shinyashiki)

SUMMARY

Metabolic syndrome (MS) can be characterized by a group of risk factors for cardiovascular disease, related to central fat distribution and insulin resistance. Obesity is growing rapidly and is directly related to MetS and some of its complications include type II diabetes *mellitus*, hypercholesterolemia and hypertension. The aim of this study is to analyze the metabolic syndrome and its relationship with pharmacotherapy. High levels of leptin and uric acid and altered fibrinolytic factors have been observed in obese individuals. Dyslipidemias are alterations in plasma lipoprotein fractions and are among the most important risk factors for atherosclerotic cardiovascular disease. Hyperinsulinemia also plays an important role in hypertension in obese individuals, as it reduces insulin sensitivity. One of the mechanisms that may explain the relationship between hyperinsulinemia and the development of hypertension is increased renal reabsorption of sodium and water. These alterations are risk factors for the development of chronic diseases such as type 2 diabetes *mellitus* and cardiovascular disease. Treatment for MetS is based mainly on lifestyle changes, for possible weight reduction and, if necessary, drug therapy to treat hypertension, diabetes *mellitus* and dyslipidemia, as these are considered risk factors for cardiovascular disease (CVD).
Keywords: Cardiovascular Disease, Diabetes *Mellitus,* Dyslipidemia, Hypertension, Obesity.

SUMMARY

1 INTRODUCTION

In 1988, Reaven described a syndrome of insulin resistance, defined as reduced glucose uptake by peripheral tissues, and called it "Syndrome X" (SALAROLI et al., 2007). It can also be called insulin resistance syndrome, lethal quartet and plurimetabolic syndrome (PAULI et al., 2006). In Brazil, the prevalence is 35.5% in people with cardiovascular disease and 8.6% in those without (BRASILEIRO-FILHO, 2011).

In epidemiological studies, the observation of populations with a low BMI that could present a high prevalence of the abnormalities characteristic of Metabolic Syndrome has raised the question that it is not the excess of total body fat, but rather the distribution of adiposity that is related to insulin resistance (I) and, consequently, to metabolic syndrome (RIBEIRO- FILHO, 2006).

Between 1986 and 1998, obesity increased by an average of 3.4% to 20% in children and adolescents, with a more atherogenic lipid profile, higher basal blood glucose levels and insulin resistance. MetS in this age group is more prevalent in obese children, who are five times more likely to develop the condition than normal individuals, and white children are three times more at risk of developing MetS than black children (BURROWS et al., 2007).

The development of MS can be genetic, due to sedentary lifestyles and smoking, where nicotine promotes the release of catecholamines, which increase heart rate, blood pressure and peripheral resistance. It also increases the body's capacity to form clots and decreases its function of destroying them. There is a reduction in oxygen in the red blood cells, because the carbon monoxide that results from burning smoke and paper binds to hemoglobin and can damage the inner wall of the vessels, leading to the deposition of fats (PESSUTO et al., 1998). Progressive weight gain due to a diet rich in refined carbohydrates, saturated fat and low in dietary fiber can also develop this syndrome (SANTOS et al., 2006).

In obese individuals, in the early stages of the disease with insulin resistance, pancreatic cells increase insulin production and secretion as a compensatory mechanism, while glucose tolerance remains normal. After some time there is a decrease in insulin secretion and consequently a decrease in glucose tolerance

(FISBERG et al., 2006).

Although it is more common in the elderly, the incidence of MS at an earlier age is increasing, especially due to lifestyle changes and the rise in obesity. The individuals most at risk of developing diabetes *mellitus* 2 are obese (MACHADO et al., 2006). Studies such as the *Bogalusa Heart Study* and the *Muscatine Study* have shown that obesity in adolescents correlates with a pro-atherogenic dyslipidemia profile, with an increase in the LDL-cholesterol fraction, increasing the cardiovascular risk already elevated by obesity (LOTTENBERG et al., 2007).

The adoption of a diet plan to reduce weight, combined with physical exercise, are considered first choice therapies for the treatment of patients with metabolic syndrome, with the expectation of reducing abdominal circumference and visceral fat, improving insulin sensitivity, reducing plasma glucose levels, and may even delay the onset of diabetes (I DIRETRIZ BRASILEIRA, 2005). The aim of this study was to analyze Metabolic Syndrome and its relationship with pharmacotherapy.

2 LITERATURE REVIEW

The proposed study is a literature review that will collect scientific information from articles, books, magazines and specific websites in the field. This information can be found in the following databases: *Pubmed, Scielo-Scientific Electronic Library Online,* Google Scholar.

This database search will use the following keywords: Metabolic Syndrome, Diabetes *Mellitus,* Dyslipidemia, Hypertension, Obesity.

For a better understanding of the subject, the work was divided into chapters. Metabolic Syndrome and Endogenous Corticoids; Inflammation in Metabolic Syndrome; The Endothelium in Metabolic Syndrome; Diagnostic Criteria for Metabolic Syndrome; Obesity in Metabolic Syndrome; Drug Treatment for Obesity; Hypertension in Metabolic Syndrome; Drug Treatment of Hypertension; Insulin Resistance and Diabetes *Mellitus* in Metabolic Syndrome; Drug Treatment of Diabetes *Mellitus*; Dyslipidemia and Atherosclerosis in Metabolic Syndrome; Drug Treatment of Dyslipidemia; Non-Drug Treatment of Metabolic Syndrome

Metabolic syndrome and endogenous corticoids

Cushing's syndrome presents glucose intolerance, insulin resistance, hypertension, dyslipidemia, central obesity, factors similar to those presented in MS, and this evidence suggests that abnormalities in the metabolism of glucocorticoids (GCs) are also associated with MS (RIBEIRO FILHO, 2006).

Some discoveries have highlighted a new mechanism of important control of the action of GCs, through the pre-receptor regulation exerted by the isoenzyme 11-beta-hydroxysteroid dehydrogenase (11^-HSD) (PAULI et al., 2006). 11^-HSDI is expressed primarily in the liver, adipocytes, kidney and brain and activates GCs, converting cortisone into cortisol at tissue level, being most active in visceral adipose tissue (RIBEIRO FILHO, 2006). 11^-HSDI plays an important role in obesity and MS, being reduced in the liver and increased in the mesenteric adipose tissue of these individuals (PAULI et al., 2006).

In skeletal muscle, high glucocorticoid activity can inhibit the insulin signaling pathway by inhibiting the translocation of GLUT4 to the cell membrane, inhibiting lipoprotein lipase and consequently reducing the uptake of triglycerides from the circulation. In liver metabolism, GCs lead to a rise in glycemia through peripheral consumption and production of glucose, stimulate liver gluconeogenesis through the release of fatty acids and glycerol from adipocytes and amino acids from inhibition of peripheral protein synthesis (PAULI et al., 2006). Specifically, GCs induce hepatocyte gluconeogenesis by activating the glucocorticoid receptors (GR) of this pathway, which stimulates the expression of phosphoenolpyruvate carboxylase and glucose-6-phosphatase, key enzymes in the gluconeogenesis cascade, resulting in increased hepatocyte glucose production and hyperglycemia (RIBEIRO FILHO, 2006).

The interaction of GCs in altering blood pressure occurs through their action on mineralocorticoid receptors, where their activation causes salt retention and a rise in blood pressure. An excess of GCs resulting from an increase in 11-3-HSD1 activity or a reduction in 11-3-HSD2 leads to activation of the MR and hypertension (PAULI *et al.*, 2006).

Inflammation in Metabolic Syndrome

Inflammation is an orderly process mediated by the appearance of intercellular adhesion molecules in the endothelium and various inflammatory mediators released by tissue cells and leukocytes. This process plays an important role in the development and progression of atherosclerosis (DUARTE et al., 2005).

Studies using cell cultures suggest that fibroblasts are the precursors of adipocytes, with the participation of extracellular signals and intrinsic transcription factors between them (LOPEZ et al., 2005). The increase in fat mass can be due to hyperplasia of adipose cells or hypertrophy of existing adipocytes. The function of the mature adipocyte will depend on its location. The subcutaneous adipocyte has different morphological and functional characteristics from the intrabdominal location. The visceral adipocyte is larger and has a greater capacity to secrete cytokines, probably associated with the characteristics of immune system cells monocytes and macrophages (BAHIA et al., 2006). Preadipocytes have the ability to phagocytize and transform into macrophage-like cells in response to certain stimuli. They also maintain the ability to differentiate throughout life, in the presence of adequate nutritional and hormonal stimuli (LOPEZ et al., 2005).

In conditions of chronic inflammation, MS is related to an increase in the blood circulation of inflammatory markers, with high plasma levels of Creactive protein (CRP), which is a pro-inflammatory cytokine (BAHIA et al., 2006), as well as interleukin 6 (IL6) and TNF-a. IL6 is correlated with body mass index (BMI) and its production is increased in visceral adipocytes. IL6 originates from immune cells, vascular stroma, endothelium and monocytes, participating as an inflammatory mediator. This mediator contributes to the increase in triglyceride concentrations in obese individuals by decreasing the production of lipoprotein lipase (LPL) and increasing the secretion of triglycerides from the liver (LOPEZ et al., 2005).

In patients with metabolic syndrome, IL6 synthesis increases along with TNF- a. TNF- a. is able to suppress LPL at the mRNA and protein level and stimulate the production of endothelin 1 and angiotensinogen in adipocytes (LOPEZ et al., 2005).

C-reactive protein, which is synthesized by the liver, has been shown in several studies to play a major role in systemic inflammation and to be capable of increasing the risk of cardiovascular disease, by stimulating IL-6 and TNF-a (FERREIRA, 2006). There is also evidence of the relationship between increased CRP concentration and increased body weight, and it has been present since childhood and adolescence, associated with the activation of endothelial cells and platelets (BAHIA et al., 2006).

After tissue damage, the presence of oxidized LDL cholesterol or an infectious agent in the vascular wall, leukocytes are activated and synthesize various cytokines, such as IL-1, IL-6 and TNF-a. IL-6 stimulates the hepatic synthesis of acute phase proteins, such as fibrinogen and C-reactive protein, where an increase in these proteins can contribute to the development of vascular events (DUARTE et al., 2005).

TNF-a. is involved in the genesis of insulin resistance by inhibiting the phosphorylation of its receptors, increasing the production of endothelin 1 and angiotensinogen, reflecting the endothelial dysfunction that can occur in obese hypertensive patients, as well as stimulating lipolysis and inhibiting lipogenesis. TNF-a is also associated with the promotion of atherosclerosis by altering platelet stability, endothelial permeability and activating monocytes and macrophages (SANTOS et al., 2006).

Metabolic syndrome is associated with an increase in fibrinogen, PAI-1 and possibly other coagulation factors, characterizing a pro-thrombotic state (I DIRETRIZ BRASILEIRA, 2005).

Increased PAI-1 concentrations promote less fibrinolytic action. In addition, there is greater production of thrombin and fibrin, due to the activation of endothelial cells, increased platelet aggregation, activation of coagulation factor VII and high concentrations of factors X, IX and prothrombin (SANTOS et al., 2006).

The endothelium in metabolic syndrome

In the last decade it has been shown that the endothelium is not simply an inert container of blood, but can be considered an endocrine organ by synthesizing and secreting various chemical mediators with multiple functions (ARPA GAMEZ et al., 2007).

The function of the endothelium is to maintain vascular homeostasis under physiological conditions, maintaining vascular tone, laminar blood flow, fluidity of the plasma membrane, balance between coagulation and fibrinolysis, inhibition of cell proliferation and migration and control of the inflammatory response. The endothelium produces nitric oxide (NO), other vasodilating substances such as endothelium-derived hyperpolarizing factor, prostacyclins and kinins and also vasoconstrictive substances such as angiotensin II and endothelin. It also produces beneficial substances, as well as NO and antioxidant factors such as the enzyme superoxide dismutase (BAHIA et al., 2006).

There is also the protective function of HDL particles, when they bind to the SR-BI (Scavenger-BI) receptor, in the active form of eNOS through the intracellular mobilization of calcium and the phosphorylation of eNOS, promoting the release of NO by endothelial cells. NO in turn has vasoactive effects which seem to be related to lysophospholipids carried by HDL and represent an anti-atherogenic function (CASELLA, 2007).

When there is an alteration in vascular relaxation due to a decrease in the bioavailability of relaxation factors derived from the endothelium, mainly NO, this is defined as endothelial dysfunction, increasing the risk of atherosclerosis. Endothelial dysfunction occurs when vasoconstrictive effects are superimposed on vasodilatory effects, generally as a result of a decrease in the bioavailability of NO, with a loss of its vasculo-protective action, generating localized inflammation and subsequently vascular lesions and thrombosis (BAHIA et al., 2006).

When an inflammatory process begins, the endothelium expresses adhesion molecules, selectins and integrins, which are capable of activating the adhesion of leukocytes to the surface of the endothelium. One of the substances that can trigger this process is the oxidation of low-density lipoprotein (LDL), which activates protein kinase C, together with a nuclear transcription factor and consequently leads to an increase in the transcription of angiotensin II, adhesion molecules and cytokines (GIGEK, 2005).

At physiological concentrations, insulin acts as a vasodilator and stimulates endothelial NO production. Glucocorticoids act antagonistically to insulin. For example, an increase in glucocorticoid production can inhibit NO synthesis by not activating eNOS, which can cause damage to the endothelium (PAULI et al., 2006).

Endothelin 1 (ET-1) is an important vasoconstrictor peptide secreted by endothelial cells in response to insulin and other agonists. In individuals with IR and atherosclerosis, high levels of ET-1 are observed. This peptide was able to inhibit insulin signaling and improve endothelium-dependent vasodilation in hyperinsulinemic rats, but had no effect in control animals. On the other hand, ET-1 also damages endothelial function by inducing NADPH-oxidase activity. Studies of endothelial function in individuals with MS who are normotolerant, intolerant or diabetic show the presence of endothelial dysfunction which worsens as glucose tolerance worsens (BAHIA et al., 2006).

At the vascular level, TNF- a. reduces the bioavailability of NO in endothelial cell culture and prevents endothelium-dependent vasodilation. Possible mechanisms suggested include a TNF-a-mediated reduction in the half-life of eNOS mRNA and an increase in superoxide production by vascular NADPH oxidase. TNF-a may also contribute to endothelial cell apoptosis (BAHIA et al., 2006).

Oxidative stress is related to endothelial dysfunction in the formation of reactive oxygen species in the vasculature, such as enzyme complexes, NADPH-oxidases and uncoupled eNOS. Elevations in NADPH-oxidase activity have been described as a result of exposure to angiotensin II and TNF-a in vascular smooth muscle cell cultures. In this process there is no decrease in NO levels, but rather an increase in its biodegradation, reducing its bioavailability (BAHIA et al., 2006). When there is superoxide in the endothelium, there is a rapid reaction with local NO, forming a reactive nitrogen species called peroxynitrite. Peroxynitrite causes direct damage to cellular DNA, as well as inducing the uncoupling of eNOS, which leads to additional production of superoxide and possible endothelial damage (SCHAAN, 2003).

There are several links between the renin-angiotensin system and vascular function: in the endothelium, the angiotensin-converting enzyme breaks down angiotensin I, produces angiotensin II and catalyzes the degradation of bradykinin, a NO-generating vasodilator. Angiotensin II stimulates the production of ET-1 and superoxide via vascular NADPH oxidase. For these and other reasons, it is necessary to inhibit this system in order to improve IR, insulin sensitivity and, consequently, endothelial function (BAHIA et al., 2006).

Diagnostic criteria for Metabolic Syndrome

According to Reaven (2006), the diagnosis of MS occurs more frequently in obese or overweight individuals, but this relationship occurs through obesity, but probably through its relationship with insulin resistance (WEARLEY, 2007).

The definitions and diagnostic proposals for MetS are described by Reaven (1988), the *World Health Organization* (WHO), the *National Cholesterol Education Program's Adult Treatment Panel* III (NCEP-ATP III) and the I Diretriz Brasileira de Diagnostico e Tratamento da Sindrome Metabolica, with concepts similar to those of the NCEP - ATP III.

The following table shows the components of the MS according to NCEP - ATP III.

Table 1 - The components of MetS according to NCEP - ATP III

COMPONENTS	
ABDOMINAL OBESITY THROUGH ABDOMINAL CIRCUMFERENCE	
Men	> 102 cm
Women	> 88 cm
TRIGLICERIDES	> 150 mg / dl

HDL - c	< 40 mg / dl
Men Women	< 50 mg / dl
BLOOD PRESSURE	> 130 mmHg or 85 mmHg
FASTING BLOOD GLUCOSE	> 110 mg / dl

An individual is characterized as having insulin resistance when he or she has a fasting blood glucose level between 100 and 126 mg/dl; above this value, diabetes is diagnosed. Insulin resistance is best determined by the homeostatic model (HOMA) (I DIRETRIZ BRASILEIRA, 2005).

Obesity in Metabolic Syndrome

The prevalence of obesity is growing all over the world and can be considered the most important nutritional disorder in developed countries, reaching 10% of this population (DUARTE et al., 2005). One of the most common ways of measuring body fat is through the body mass index (BMI), with BMI above 30 kg/m^2 . An accumulation of energy in the form of fat in adipose tissue can raise blood pressure, increase the risk of cardiovascular disease and alter the lipid profile (VALDELAMAR et al., 2007).

In a previous study of British women, Regidor et al. observed the cumulative effect of adverse socio-economic circumstances during childhood and adulthood on various components of MS. Due to physical inactivity, they were more likely to become obese, a major risk factor for the onset of MS (REGIDOR et al., 2007).

There are two types of fat distribution, the lower or hip type and the upper central type, android, with distribution at the level of the trunk, with increased deposition in the visceral intra-abdominal region, which has a faster *turnover* than other regions, increasing concentrations of plasminogen activator inhibitor-1 (PAI-1), inflammatory cytokines and non-esterified fatty acids in the portal system (SANTOS et al., 2006).

The accumulation of fat in the muscles leads to insulin resistance, while in the liver it promotes atherogenic dyslipidemia (SANTOS et al., 2006). In addition, it can lead to the appearance of target diseases such as diabetes *mellitus,* systemic arterial hypertension, dyslipidemia, certain forms of cancer and osteoarthritis, among others

(MANCINI et al., 2006). Morbid obesity is a state of insulin resistance associated with excess visceral fat, conditions that contribute to the development of MS (GELONEZE et al., 2006), increasing the risk of cardiometabolic problems (CASELLA, 2007).

In obesity, insulin secretion is increased, while hepatocyte uptake and peripheral insulin efficacy decrease (MCLELLAN et al., 2006). This decreases the hepatic extraction of insulin, contributing to systemic hyperinsulinemia and future insulin resistance (FERREIRA, 2006).

Obesity and physical activity levels are powerful mediators of insulin-mediated glucose availability, and in contrast to other factors that affect insulin action, they are modifiable by lifestyle changes (DUARTE et al., 2005). Glucose in skeletal muscle is also stimulated by insulin-independent mechanisms, which are activated by hypoxia, nitric oxide and bradykinin (PAULI et al., 2006).

Studies have shown that a significant increase in body weight is associated with greater sympathetic activation. Individuals with a waist-to-hip ratio greater than 1.0 have significantly higher pulse pressure and heart rate, which also correlates with increased excretion of catecholamine metabolites, as well as unfavorable glycemia, insulinemia and lipid profile (MATOS et al., 2003).

Increased SNS activity could not only be responsible for the rise in blood pressure and heart rate, but also for the increased mobilization of free fatty acids (FFA) from adipose tissue. Elevated fatty acid levels are an important finding in abdominal obesity, exerting profound peripheral effects on the development of insulin resistance in the muscles and liver (BAHIA et al., 2006).

There is evidence that FFA reduce the bioavailability of nitric oxide (NO) (MATOS et al., 2003) by inhibiting the activity of the enzyme nitric oxide synthase (eNOS) and stimulating the production of reactive oxygen species by NADPH oxidase (BAHIA et al., 2006).

Obesity is a state of relative hypo-somatotropism, with a decreased GH response to various known stimuli. The amount of adipose tissue is directly related to plasma FFA levels, which are higher in patients with central-visceral obesity, and acute or chronic increases in FFA are capable of inhibiting GH release by the pituitary gland. Casanueva et al. demonstrated that the addition of oleic and caprylic acid to somatotrophic cells in vitro is capable of inducing a direct blockade of GH release (MATOS et al., 2003).

With the discovery of leptin in 1994, the endocrine function of adipocytes was confirmed, and a large number of hormone-acting peptides were also discovered which regulate energy expenditure, the feeling of satiety and participate in macronutrient metabolism. Leptin expression and secretion are stimulated by insulin, glucocorticoids, TNF-a and estrogens and inhibited by beta adrenergic activity, androgens, free fatty acids, growth hormone and PPAR-6 agonists. Its effects on energy intake and expenditure are mediated by hypothalamic pathways. In the cardiovascular system, leptin acts at different levels, increasing sympathetic discharge, insulin resistance and sodium and water excretion (LOPEZ DE FEZ et al., 2004).

Adiponectin, whose messenger RNA is expressed exclusively in adipose tissue, maintains plasma concentrations inversely proportional to body fat mass, especially in cases of visceral obesity (LOPEZ et al., 2005). It has anti-inflammatory, anti-atherogenic and insulin-sensitizing effects and participates in the regulation of energy homeostasis, working in combination with leptin. It also has a direct effect on the vasculature, through increased phosphorylation of eNOS, increased production of NO and inhibition of TNF-a, as well as indirect beneficial effects (BAHIA et al., 2006). There is a reduction in adiponectin expression in individuals with diabetes, coronary heart disease and hypertension (LOPEZ et al., 2005).

Exercise in obese patients has an effect on weight loss by increasing the activity of the hormone-sensitive enzyme lipase and increasing mitochondrial density, boosting lipid oxidation and consequently reducing body weight (PAULI et al., 2006).

Drug Treatment for Obesity

Pharmacological treatment for obesity is an area of sudden change and the development of new products and proposals. In MS patients, treatment is indicated for those who have been unable to reduce their weight through diet and exercise alone. The aim of drug treatment is to produce an energy deficit by utilizing the body's energy reserves and reducing caloric intake, leading to weight loss and an improved metabolic profile (VALDELAMAR et al., 2007).

The following drugs have been registered in Brazil for drug treatment: Sibutramine and Orlistat (I DIRETRIZ BRASILEIRA, 2005).

The choice of an anti-obesity drug should also be based on the individual's previous experience and previous use of medication, although the failure of a previous treatment does not justify not using a particular agent afterwards (MANCINI et a ., 2006).

Among these experiences, some criteria have been established for anti-obesity drug therapy, such as:

1. Pharmacological treatment is only justified in conjunction with dietary advice ard lifestyle changes. Pharmacological agents only help to increase patients' adherence to nutritional and behavioral changes.
2. When discontinued, drug treatment does not cure obesity; weight regain occurs. Like any other treatment in medicine, drugs don't work when they're not taken, i.e. you should expect to regain the weight you've lost when you stop taking them.
3. Anti-obesity drugs should be used under continuous medical supervision.
4. The treatment and choice of medication is tailored to each patient. The risks associated with the use of a drug must be weighed against the risks of persistent obesity.
5. Treatment should only be continued when it is considered safe and effective for the patient in question (MANCINI et al., 2006).

The most widely used criteria for evaluating the effectiveness of anti-obesity treatments are those of the FDA *(Food and* Drug *Administration)* (LOFEZ et al., 2005) and the CPMP *(Committee of the European Agency for the Evaluation of Medicinal Products)* (MANCINI et al., 2006).

Fluctuating weight, commonly observed in long-term treatments, has the basic characteristic of a cycle consisting of intentional weight loss and unirtentional weight gain, which interferes with the improvement of risk factors present in MS (ANDRADE et al., 2004).

Orlistat

Lipstatin is a compound produced by a fungus, *Streptomyces toxytricini.* Orlistat is a more stable and partially hydrolyzed analogue of lipstatin. It is a specific inhibitor of pancreatic lipase, the enzyme that catalyzes the hydrolytic remova of triglycerides from food (MENDIVIL, 2005).

The use of orlistat in therapeutic doses (120 mg) inhibits the digestion of 30% of dietary triglycerides. Orlistat binds irreversibly to the active site of lipase through covalent bonding. Around a third of the triglycerides ingested remain undigested and are not absorbed by the small intestine, passing through the GI tract and being eliminated in the feces (MANCINI et al., 2006), thus reducing the increase in calories from food. Because it is not absorbed into the bloodstream, orlistat can have side effects such as oily stools, an increase in the number of bowel movements, flatulence with or without the elimination of fat, and fecal urgency. Orlistat is the only drug for the treatment of obesity that has a controlled clinical trial study lasting more than four years. Orlistat therapy produces a significant reduction in waist circumference, systolic and diastolic blood pressure, LDL cholesterol, improved insulinemia and glucose tolerance (MENDIVIL, 2005).

Orlistat has no effect on appetite-regulating neuronal circuits. However, the pharmacological effect of orlistat, evidenced by the amount of fat in the feces, stimulates long-term adherence to eating foods with a lower fat content (MANCINI et al., 2006).

Efficacy of Orlistat in patients with metabolic syndrome

In some studies, Dr. Reaven evaluated the treatment of obesity in patients with metabolic syndrome, resulting in significant reductions in body weight (8.5 kg) and LDL cholesterol (9.5 mg/dl) (MENDIVIL, 2005). The mechanism by which orlistat lowers the LDL-c value is based on inhibiting the absorption of triglycerides from food, with the fatty acids from these triglycerides being the main substrate for the liver's synthesis of cholesterol. The reason for not reducing VLDL-c particles is that these particles transport endogenous triglycerides, where orlistat has no action (MENDIVIL, 2005).

Sibutramine

Sibutramine is a drug that was initially developed with antidepressant potential and works as a specific inhibitor of noradrenaline and serotonin reuptake in the nerve endings of the sympathetic system at central and peripheral level. It also stimulates the release of catecholamines, being a direct agonist (MENDIVIL, 2005).

The antagonism of serotonin 5HT receptors and beta-1 adrenergic receptors at a central level promotes appetite suppression and prolongs satiety, while at a peripheral level it has a slight effect by increasing thermogenesis, increasing the metabolic rate and increasing energy expenditure, due to the activation of beta3 adrenergic receptors in fat tissue (ARAUJO et al., 2000).

Sibutramine prevents the decrease in basal metabolic rate that is suggested as the body's response to weight loss (MENDIVIL, 2005). It also has thermogenic properties, affecting the energy balance by increasing the metabolic rate via the adrenergic receptor (HALPERN et al., 2000).

Sibutramine acts on the plasma membrane receptors at the post-synaptic nerve endings, which would be activated by serotonin. Sibutramine activates them, triggering a signaling cascade, characterized by the activation of the G-coupled protein, thus increasing the concentrations of cyclic AMP. This is followed by the activation of the enzyme phospholipase A, with an increase in the second messenger Inositol 3-phosphate (IP3), resulting in the expression of genes coding for and inhibiting the release of neuropeptide Y, which is an orexigenic agent (VALDELAMAR et al., 2007).

Sibutramine has a central action, but no adipose potential, as it does not affect the dopaminergic reward circuits, as is the case with amphetamines and manzidol. There have also been no reports of pulmonary hypertension (MENDIVIL, 2005).

Effectiveness of Sibutramine in patients with metabolic syndrome

Treatment with sibutramine in two-year clinical trials reported significant reductions in body weight of 5 to 6 kg, with no relationship to the dose (MENDIVIL, 2005). Sibutramine reduces food intake and also stimulates thermogenesis in brown adipose tissue in experimental animals (MANCINI et al., 2006).

Although there have been no trials in patients with metabolic syndrome, treatment has been associated with positive changes in waist circumference and HDL in several studies, as well as improvements in metabolic control in obese patients with type 2 diabetes. Sibutramine therapy can raise blood pressure and resting heart rate

(MENDIVIL, 2005). Anticholinergic effects such as dry mouth, headache, constipation, insomnia or drowsiness, rhinitis and pharyngitis may also occur (HALPERN et al., 2002).

Associations of two pharmacological agents

Although there are no randomized studies on the combination of sibutramine and orlistat, it has been used in clinical practice to treat obese patients, since the site of action of these drugs is different. The association of sibutramine and orlistat in the treatment of obesity, in a study in private clinics, promoted a much greater weight reduction than that reported in randomized clinical studies and the tolerability of the association was very reasonable (MANCINI et al., 2006).

Hypertension in Metabolic Syndrome

Blood pressure is the perfusion of arterial blood per minute, cardiac output, and the vascular or peripheral resistance imposed on this flow. It results from the interaction of cardiac work, through the action of contraction and relaxation of the cardiac muscles, and the elastic property of the blood vessels (FERREIRA, 2006).

Hypertension is a multifactorial clinical entity in which high blood pressure levels, metabolic and hormonal alterations and trophic phenomena are present. Blood pressure is determined by the product of cardiac output and peripheral vascular resistance, varying physiologically with various factors such as state of vigilance, physical activity, drug use, respiratory movements, among others (DUARTE et al., 2005).

Hyperinsulinemia also plays an important role in the development of hypertension in obese individuals, due to the deterioration of insulin sensitivity in peripheral tissues (FERREIRA, 2006). The mechanisms that may explain this relationship are increased renal reabsorption of sodium and water, activation of the sympathetic nervous system, hormones associated with high triglyceride levels

(FARIA et al., 2002).

Sodium retention is caused by decreased sodium elimination. The vasoconstrictive action of the SNS in skeletal muscle vessels reduces glucose absorption by the muscle, favoring insulin resistance and hyperinsulinemia. The increase in intracellular calcium in smooth muscle cells is due to a decrease in Na-K ATPase, which can lead to hypertension, increased muscle tone and peripheral resistance (LOPEZ DE FEZ et al., 2004).

Increased blood pressure is directly related to increased consumption of sodium, alcohol and smoking, and inversely to the use of foods rich in potassium, calcium and magnesium (DUARTE et al., 2005). It is also directly related to obesity, where serum concentrations of angiotensinogen are increased due to its greater synthesis by adipocytes, thus generating more angiotensin II and consequently raising blood pressure (SANTOS et al., 2006).

The renin-angiotensin system is a blood pressure control system. It can be activated by various stimuli, and after this activation, the kidney releases a large quantity of renin, a proteolytic enzyme, which acts on the angiotensinogen, releasing angiotensin I. This decapeptide has little hemodynamic or metabolic effect and can be transformed by a dipeptidase, the angiotensin I-converting enzyme, into angiotensin II. Angiotensin II produces various effects such as arteriolar contraction, increases the secretion of aldosterone, resulting in a decrease in glomerular filtration, and increases the secretion of vasopressin and ACTH. These and other effects of angiotensin II can contribute to an increase in blood pressure (SANTOS et al., 2006).

Drug treatment for hypertension

Metabolic syndrome has several cardiovascular risk factors, and in most cases drug treatment is necessary to prevent these risks and to prevent metabolic deterioration. For the treatment of arterial hypertension, the drug should be evaluated according to certain principles, such as being effective orally, well tolerated by the patient at the lowest possible dose, considering combined use with other drugs and also evaluating the patient's socio-economic conditions (I DIRETRIZ BRASILEIRA, 2005).

The therapeutic decision must also take into account, in addition to blood pressure values, the presence or absence of target organ damage and associated cardiovascular risk factors (KOHLMANN, 1999).

Blood pressure is treated with lifestyle changes, physical activity, reducing body weight and restricting salt in the diet, with or without the use of medication, which can also be administered alone or in combination (BRUNTON et al., 2006).

Patients with target organ damage or clinically identifiable cardiovascular disease or diabetes *mellitus* are recommended immediate pharmacological treatment, in addition to non-pharmacological treatment (MION et al., 2001).

A model therapeutic regimen for the treatment of hypertension in patients with metabolic syndrome is based initially on modifying the individual's lifestyle. If no reduction in blood pressure is achieved, monotherapy is used, looking at the causes of the rise in blood pressure (BRUNTON et al., 2006).

If blood pressure does not reach the desired levels, the dose of the drug should be increased to the maximum permitted. If the target levels are still not reached, one or more classes of drugs can be associated with each other as long as there is a proven benefit of this association in reducing the patient's cardiovascular risk, and the subsequent steps are to optimize the doses of these drugs (CORREA et al., 2006).

Drug combinations should be based on the premise of not combining drugs with similar mechanisms of action, with the exception of combining thiazide diuretics and potassium-sparing algae. For cases of hypertension resistant to dual therapy, therapy with three or more drugs can be prescribed. In this situation, the use of diuretics is essential (KOHLMANN, 1999).

Angiotensin Converting Enzyme Inhibitors (ACEI)

The mechanism of action of these substances is fundamentally dependent on the inhibition of the converting enzyme, thus blocking the transformation of angiotensin I into II in the blood and tissues. They are effective as monotherapy in the treatment of hypertension (KOHLMANN, 1999).

Treatment with ACE inhibitors reduces cardiovascular morbidity and mortality in patients with MS and slows the decline in renal function in patients with diabetic nephropathy. Monitoring serum potassium levels is indicated to assess declining renal function, since hyperkalemia is a frequent cause of ACEI discontinuation in diabetic patients with nephropathy (FARIA et al., 2002).

These hypotensive drugs have no harmful effects on lipid and glucose metabolism (I DIRETRIZ BRASILEIRA, 2005). In association with diuretics, the antihypertensive action of ACE inhibitors is increased and postural hypotension may occur (KOHLMANN, 1999; FARIA et al., 2002).

ACE inhibitors act synergistically with diuretics and calcium channel blockers and can even lower lipids by improving carbohydrate metabolism. The mechanism of action for improving glucose utilization may involve the generation of kinins by ACEIs. One possible explanation could be that the increase in blood flow determined by the increase in kinins would lead to better insulin release and greater glucose uptake by the tissues (FARIA et al., 2002).

ACE inhibitors are beneficial for obese patients because they increase insulin sensitivity, improve endothelial function by decreasing angiotensin II and consequently decreasing the generation of free radicals from NADPH-oxidase, increasing bradykinin and NO (NEUTEL, 2004), which are possible mechanisms involved in the cardioprotective effects of ACE inhibitors (FARIA et al., 2002).

The use of captopril in animals subjected to salt restriction was able to improve their sensitivity to insulin, while the inhibition of ATI receptors with losartan did not show the same effect, suggesting that the effect of the drug could be the result of an increase in bradykinin rather than the actual inhibition of the effects of angiotensin II, predicting that these mechanisms may involve key steps in insulin signaling (MACHADO et al., 2006).

Undesirable effects include dry cough, altered taste and hypersensitivity reactions such as rash and edema. In individuals with chronic renal failure, they can induce hyperpotassemia (KOHLMANN, 1999).

Angiotensin II receptor antagonists (ARA-II)

These drugs antagonize the action of angiotensin II by specifically blocking its ATI receptors. They are effective as monotherapy in the treatment of hypertensive patients. They have a good tolerability profile and the side effects reported are dizziness and, rarely, rash (KOHLMANN, 1999).

Angiotensin II receptor antagonists can be used to treat the increase in blood pressure in patients with metabolic syndrome. These drugs have advantages over other treatments when it comes to the process of atherosclerosis and cardiovascular risk because they act in two ways, firstly via the PPARgamma pathway, reducing insulin resistance, dyslipidemia and inflammation and also via the angiotensin II pathway, reducing cell proliferation, hypertension and oxidation (MOLINA, 2005), proving effective in preventing nephropathy and cardiovascular protection in type 2 diabetic individuals (FARIA et al., 2002).

In hypertensive type 2 diabetic patients, according to *Irbesartan in Microalbuminuria of Type 2 Diabetes* (IRMA2), angiotensin II blockade, regardless of its antihypertensive action, is effective in preventing the progression of kidney disease from the albuminuric phase to the proteinuric phase, as well as delaying the evolution from the proteinuric phase to the final stages of kidney disease, in addition to providing cardiovascular protection (FARIA et al., 2002).

ATI receptor blockers are also capable of reducing the production of superoxide ions at the level of the endothelium and vascular smooth muscle, consequently increasing the bioavailability of NO and limiting the oxidation of LDL molecules (BAHIA et al., 2006).

Diuretics

Individuals with metabolic syndrome have various mechanisms that induce sodium retention, so the use of a diuretic is necessary. The use of thiazide diuretics is recommended (IDIRETRIZ BRASILEIRA, 2005). In clinical practice, it is almost impossible to control blood pressure in diabetics without the use of diuretics. It is often necessary to replace thiazides with alpha-diuretics in order to achieve blood pressure control, especially when kidney damage has progressed (FARIA et al., 2002).

The antihypertensive mechanism of diuretics is related to the increased excretion of sodium and water by the body, through an action on the kidneys. Their primary effect consists of decreasing the reabsorption of sodium and chloride from the filtrate, while the increase in water loss is secondary to the increased excretion of salt and consequent reduction in peripheral vascular resistance due to various mechanisms (PELLIZZARO et al., 2003).

Potassium-sparing diuretics have little diuretic potency, but when combined with thiazides and alpa diuretics they are useful in the prevention and treatment of hypopotassemia. The use of potassium-sparing diuretics in patients with reduced renal function can lead to hyperpotassemia. The undesirable effects of diuretics include hypopotassemia and hyperuricemia. The fact that
diuretics can cause glucose intolerance. They can also cause an increase in serum triglyceride levels, which is generally dose-dependent. In many cases, they cause sexual dysfunction. In general, the appearance of the undesirable effects of diuretics is related to the dosage used. Diuretics should be used with caution in patients with MS, as they can increase insulin resistance and lead to glucose intolerance (KOHLMANN, 1999).

Calcium channel antagonists

Calcium channel antagonists act by blocking the entry of calcium in response to depolarization; they dilate the capacitance resistance vessels (PELLIZZARO et al., 2003).

They are effective in the treatment of hypertension and do not cause changes in lipid and carbohydrate metabolism, but their long-term effects in relation to the progression of diabetic nephropathy have not yet been established (GALVAO et al., 2002).

Calcium channel blockers do not seem to be as effective in preventing coronary heart disease as ACE inhibitors (FARIA et al., 2002).

The adverse effects of this group include headache, dizziness, facial flushing and peripheral edema. More rarely, they can induce gingival hypertrophy. Verapamil and diltiazem can cause myocardial depression and atrioventricular block (KOHLMANN, 1999).

They are the first-choice drugs for the treatment of hypertension associated with coronary artery disease (I DIRECTRIZ BRASILEIRA, 2005).

The antihypertensive mechanism, which is complex, involves a reduction in cardiac output, in the initial action, a reduction in renin secretion, readaptation of the baroreceptors and a reduction in cardiovascular morbidity and mortality.

These drugs have restrictions for use in patients with MS, because from a metabolic point of view, they can induce weight gain, glucose intolerance, insulin resistance, hypertriglyceridemia and a reduction in HDL-c, as well as a lower capacity to perform physical exercise (FARIA et al., 2002).

Undesirable reactions to beta-blockers include bronchospasm, excessive bradycardia, atrioventricular conduction disorders, myocardial depression, peripheral vasoconstriction, insomnia, nightmares, psychic depression, asthenia and sexual dysfunction. Abrupt discontinuation of these blockers can cause sympathetic hyperactivity, with rebound hypertension or manifestations of myocardial ischemia. Beta-blockers are formally contraindicated in patients with asthma, chronic obstructive pulmonary disease and atrioventricular block. They should be used with caution in patients with peripheral arterial obstructive disease (KOHLMANN, 1999).

Insulin Resistance and Diabetes *Mellitus* in Metabolic Syndromes

Diabetes *mellitus* is a syndrome characterized by elevated fasting blood glucose, caused by a relative or absolute deficiency of insulin, or by a reduction in the sensitivity of the tissues to this hormone. Diabetes is characterized by polyuria, polydipsia, weight loss, although it induces increased appetite and hyperglycemia. This pathology has a large amount of glucose in the interstitial space and a lack of glucose in the intracellular space, generating a situation known as "hunger in the midst of plenty of food" (HEIMANN, 2003).

In type 2 diabetes *mellitus* and impaired glucose tolerance, resistance to insulin-stimulated glucose uptake is observed, regardless of hyperglycemia, and the deterioration of this tolerance will depend on the pancreas' ability to maintain the state of chronic hyperinsulinemia (MCLELLAN et al., 2006). In obese individuals, in the early stages of the disease, due to insulin resistance, the pancreatic β-cells increase insulin production and secretion as a compensatory mechanism^, while glucose tolerance is normal, then there is a decline in insulin secretion and, consequently, a decrease in glucose tolerance, which can lead the individual to develop type 2 diabetes *mellitus* and cardiovascular disease (FERREIRA, 2006).

In this process, alterations occur in the metabolism of macronutrients, leading to a predominance of tissue catabolism. Diabetes affects almost 200 million people worldwide and is the fourth leading cause of death in the world (LOMBO et al., 2007). It is characterized as a metabolic disease with serious implications for patients' quality of life due to its microvascular and macrovascular complications (CASTRO et al., 2006). Among the metabolic alterations in diabetes *mellitus,* there is a phenotype of inappropriate hyperglycemia. Chronic hyperglycemia is accompanied by dyslipidemia, hypertension and endothelial dysfunction, both risk factors in MS (DUARTE et al , 2005).

Insulin resistance is the inability of insulin to produce biological effects at normal concentrations, which may be related to a deficiency in the insulin receptor or a defect in some post-receptor mechanism (DUARTE et al., 2005). It occurs when the normal concentration of this hormone produces a lower biological response in peripheral tissues such as muscle, liver and adipose tissue. The activation of the insulin receptor results in the translocation of the GLUT4 protein from the cytosol to the cell membrane, which allows glucose to enter the cell. Resistance can also occur when there is a reduction in the amount of GLUT4 or in the translocation of GLUT4 to the membrane, which is considered to be the most important factor (SANTOS et al., 2006).

This reduction in expression can occur in adipose tissue and is associated with IR, regardless of the regulation that occurs in skeletal muscle. Researchers have shown that, during the process of developing obesity, initially, when weight gain is accelerated, there is an increase in insulin sensitivity and GLUT4 in adipose tissue, later, when obesity stabilizes, there is a reduction in GLUT4 in adipose tissue and IR manifests itself (MACHADO et al., 2006).

Insulin resistance is particularly linked to obesity, as adipose tissue has the capacity to secrete substances with important biological effects that act both locally (paracrine effects) and systemically (endocrine effects) (MCLELLAN et al., 2006).

The mechanism that justifies this hypothesis focuses on free fatty acids, provided by lipolysis, which in the long term lead to a decrease in peripheral glucose utilization and inhibit insulin secretion by в cells, leading to lipotoxicity, which may be the genesis of diabetes *mellitus* 2 (FERREIRA, 2006). The mechanism involves an increase in NO production and the synthesis of inflammatory cytokines and polypeptides, such as leptin, resistin, PAI-1, TNF-a and IL-6, except for adiponectin, which is decreased by this process (MCLELLAN et al., 2006). Monocytes adhered to adipose tissue differentiate into macrophages, which produce the same cytokines, thus increasing the inflammatory response. An increase in the supply of circulating free fatty acids, oxidative stress, hypertension and an increase in small, dense LDL molecules are some of the possible mechanisms involved in the lower supply of NO resulting from insulin resistance (BAHIA et al., 2006).

In a study carried out by Pivatto and his colleagues, it was shown that insulin resistance, an index obtained by the hemostatic assessment model (HOMA-IR), is the most prevalent risk factor for MetS and the proinsulin/insulin index showed no significant association with MetS. According to the HOMA-IR results, proinsulin and insulin showed good negative predictive values, which could be used to identify a population at risk (PIVATTO et al., 2007).

According to studies published by Atala (2006), increased intra-abdominal fat in individuals with type 1 diabetes *mellitus* was related to an atherosclerotic lipid profile similar to that observed in individuals without diabetes but with MS (ATALA, 2006). Chronic hyperglycemia can lead to alterations in the GLUT-2 glucose transporters located in the в-cells and a reduction in the amount of GLUT-4 in muscle tissue (FERREIRA, 2006). These processes lead to a decrease in insulin sensitivity, which in turn reduces the severity of kidney function (ATALA, 2006).

Drug Treatment for Diabetes Mellitus

Treatment for this risk factor in metabolic syndrome should aim to regulate and maintain blood glucose levels.

Oral antidiabetics

Oral antidiabetics act by reducing the rate of absorption of glycerides (alpha-glucose inhibitors), reducing the hepatic production of glucose (biguanides), increasing its peripheral utilization (glycotazones) and increasing the pancreatic secretion of insulin (sulphonylureas and glinides). Among the antihyperglycemic drugs, metformin stands out for its mechanism of reducing hepatic glucose production, with less peripheral sensitizing action. Glitazones also act more on peripheral insulin resistance in muscle, fat cells and hepatocytes, making them an excellent ally in the hyperglycemic treatment of MS patients (I DIRETRIZ BRASILEIRA, 2005).

The choice of drug will depend on fasting and postprandial glycemia values, glycated hemoglobin, weight, age, complications and associated diseases. To lower blood glucose, two or more oral anti-diabetics with different mechanisms of action can be combined. In the event of an inadequate response, the introduction of insulin to the drug combination is indicated (I DIRETRIZ BRASILEIRA, 2005).

Metformin

Metformin was extracted from a medicinal herb, which has hypoglycemic properties, but its mechanism of action is not yet fully understood. In a study by the *Diabetes Prevention Program Research Group,* it was shown that both the administration of metformin and changes in lifestyle, diet and physical exercise, reduced the incidence of type 2 diabetes *mellitus* when compared to the control group. The study also showed that both metformin and rigorous lifestyle changes were able to significantly reduce fasting blood glucose and the percentage of glycated hemoglobin (KNOWLER, 2006).

This result may not just be coincidental, as it has recently been shown that AMPK, which is stimulated by physical exercise, is also possibly the target of metformin's action. AMPK is a sensitizer of the cellular energy balance and is activated by an increase in the AMP/ATP ratio. AMPK is a probable target of metformin and there are indications that it is responsible for beneficial effects in the treatment and prevention of type 2 diabetes *mellitus* and metabolic syndrome (SANTOMAURO et al., 2008).

This biguanide reduces blood glucose by increasing the number and improving the affinity of insulin receptors, both in the adipocyte and in the muscle (ARAUJO et al., 2000), mainly by hepatocyte and muscle agonists that have an insulin-sensitizing effect. It inhibits gluconeogenesis and glycogenolysis, and stimulates glycogenolysis in the hepatocyte, and in insulin-dependent peripheral tissues, especially skeletal muscle, it increases glucose uptake, causing a rapid reduction in plasma glucose (SANTOMAURO et al., 2008).

In the adipocyte, metformin inhibits lipolysis and the availability of free fatty acids, can reduce LDL-cholesterol and promote a slight increase in HDL-c, improves endothelial function, with a decrease in PAI-1 (ARAUJO et al., 2000), causes a slight reduction in blood pressure and reduces weight in individuals with diabetes or peripheral insulin resistance, possibly due to its anorexigenic properties (SANTOMAURO et al., 2008). At the cellular level, metformin increases the activity of insulin receptor tyrosine kinase, stimulating GLUT4 translocation and glycogen synthase activity (ARAUJO, et al. 2000).

The studies by Zang et al. showed that AMPK activation is necessary for metformin to exert its lipid-lowering effects. This occurs through the phosphorylation and consequent inactivation of ACC and HMGCoA reductase in hepatocytes, contributing to a reduction in the content of fatty acids and cholesterol, as well as decreasing the synthesis of lipoproteins. As a consequence of this effect, there is an increase in fatty acid oxidation in the hepatocyte, reducing hepatocyte steatosis and improving the liver's sensitivity to insulin (SANTOMAURO et al., 2008).

Metformin has the potential to reduce cardiovascular risk in diabetes *mellitus* 2, by activating the AMPK enzyme, and should be further evaluated in the context of metabolic syndrome, as it has favorable effects on body weight and plasma lipids, for these reasons metformin can be considered the first choice for treatment in obese people with type 2 diabetes *mellitus* (MARTIN MUNOZ et al., 2005).

Monotherapy with metformin is indicated for obese or even glucose intolerant diabetics. The use of metformin is associated with less weight gain, a lower incidence of hypoglycemia and lower plasma insulin levels (FARIA et al., 2002). When satisfactory control is not achieved, it can be used in association with sulfonylurea, acarbose, thiazolidinedione, repaglinide and/or insulin. The most common side effects are diarrhea, metallic taste and nausea, which sometimes subside with continued use of the medication. Decreased absorption of vitamin B12 has been described (ARAUJO et al., 2000).

Rosiglitazone

PPAR- g receptors are part of a family of nuclear receptors that are expressed mainly in adipose tissue, but also in vascular endothelial cells, macrophages and pancreatic beta cells. Thiazolidinediones (TZDs) are their exogenous agonists and are potent sensitizers of insulin action. These substances have therefore been used in the treatment of type 2 diabetes *mellitus* with the aim of improving IR through direct effects on adipose tissue, increasing the uptake of fatty acids and glucose, they increase the expression of glucose transporters (GLUT4) and indirectly, by altering the secretion of adipocytokines, by decreasing TNF-a and increasing adiponectin, increasing the expression of lipoprotein lipase, reducing the expression of leptin (ARAUJO et al., 2000) and consequently improve insulin sensitivity in other tissues.

Rosiglitazone has effects on glucose metabolism, demonstrates a potent anti-inflammatory action and, in diabetic patients, was able to significantly improve endothelial function. Thus, early intervention with this agent in non-diabetic patients with MS could help improve endothelial function, and its anti-inflammatory action could improve the cardiovascular risk of these patients (BAHIA et al., 2006).

It is possible that thiazolidinediones reduce the progression of atherosclerosis, since in rats subjected to arterial injury, troglitazone inhibited the growth of vascular smooth muscle cells and intimal hyperplasia. In diabetics treated with troglitazone, decreases in platelet adhesion, PAI-1 and blood pressure levels were observed. These multiple effects strengthen its indication in the treatment of metabolic syndrome (ARAUJO et al., 2000).

Bahia and his colleagues, in their study of the effects of rosiglitazone on endothelial function in non-diabetic individuals with metabolic syndrome, showed that the patients analyzed using rosiglitazone had increased body weight; the women deposited fat in the peripheral region, with an increase in hip measurement and a decrease in waist-to-hip ratio. With regard to the lipid profile, there was an increase in total cholesterol, LDL-cholesterol and, only in the female group, an increase in HDL-cholesterol.

It also induced a reduction in IR, fibrinogen and CRP and improved endothelial function in individuals with MS. These data suggest a possible role for this substance in regulating endothelial function. The prophylactic use of TZDs in individuals at high risk of developing diabetes and cardiovascular disease (those with metabolic syndrome and glucose intolerance) has not yet been established (BAHIA et al., 2006).

Treatment with thiazolidinediones can be used as monotherapy or in association with metformin, with which it has a potentiated antihyperglycemic effect, or with sulfonylurea, meglitinide or even insulin, especially in diabetics with metabolic syndrome. The combination of thiazolidinedione with metformin is interesting because it has additive effects (ARAUJO et al., 2000).

Side effects can include upper respiratory tract infections, headaches, elevated transaminases, edema, weight gain and anemia. An FDA review of adverse reactions found cases of significant weight gain and edema, both signs of heart failure (ARAUJO et al., 2000).

Sulfonylureas

The choice of type of sulphonylurea depends on the patient's age, tolerability and response to the medication. [a]There are first-generation sulphonylureas such as chlorpropamide, second-generation sulphonylureas such as glibenclamide, glicazide and glipizide, and third-generation sulphonylureas such as glimepiride (ARAUJO et al., 2000).

The mechanism of action of these drugs on the pancreatic beta cell when stimulated by hyperglycemia is the regulation of KATP channels. At the cellular level, sulfonylureas act by inhibiting KATP channels, depolarizing the pancreatic beta cell and stimulating calcium influx and insulin secretion. They can also act in the short term by increasing insulin secretion, or by increasing the number of insulin receptors and having a post-receptor effect, facilitating insulin support (RANG, 2011).

Alpha-glucosidase inhibitors

The competitive alpha-glucosidase inhibitors, acarbose, miglitol and voglibose, act as enzyme antagonists of amylase and sucrase and reduce the intestinal absorption of glucose (ARAUJO et al., 2000). These drugs do not interfere with insulin secretion and reduce fasting glycemia and postprandial hyperglycemia.

The most common side effects are flatulence, diarrhea, abdominal pain and elevated transaminases. Acarbose can be combined with another oral antidiabetic or insulin. Triglyceride levels may decrease with the use of miglitol (ARAUJO et al., 2000).

Acarbose can be used as an alternative treatment or in patients who will modify their lifestyle, to delay the development of type 2 diabetes *mellitus* in patients with impaired glucose tolerance (MCLELLAN et al., 2006).

Insulin

Insulin therapy in type 2 diabetes *mellitus* is reserved for symptomatic diabetics with severe hyperglycemia, with ketonemia or ketonuria, even if they have just been diagnosed, or for diabetics who do not respond to treatment with diet, exercise and/or oral hypoglycemic agents, antihyperglycemic agents or insulin action sensitizers. The combination of insulin and oral hypoglycemic agents seems to be beneficial in some cases. In those patients who have postprandial hyperglycemia, the use of metformin, acarbose, repaglinide or nateglinide can improve the glycemic profile, reduce the insulin dose and minimize weight gain (ARAUJO et al., 2000).

In some cases, therapy with sulphonylureas or insulin has been associated with clinically undesirable effects such as high plasma insulin levels, increased body weight and a greater risk of hypoglycaemia (MARTIN MUNOZ et al., 2005).

Dyslipidemia and Atherosclerosis in Metabolic Syndromes

Plasma lipoproteins are lipid-carrying vehicles in the circulation. They are macromolecular complexes that are slightly soluble in water and have the function of transporting triglycerides and cholesterol from their place of origin to storage and use as an energy source. In humans there is a large deposition of lipids, especially cholesterol, in the tissues, which poses a great risk due to the formation of plaques, which cause narrowing of the blood vessels and can result in atherosclerosis.

VLDL-c is the main carrier of endogenous triglycerides, which are hydrolyzed in extrahepatic tissues by lipoprotein lipase (LPL) and the remaining particles are metabolized by the liver. LDL-c carries cholesterol to the peripheral tissues, half of which is degraded by the liver and the other half by extrahepatic tissues (FERREIRA, 2006).

Dyslipidemia is an alteration in the function of plasma lipoproteins and is one of the most important risk factors for atherosclerotic cardiovascular disease and is part of a group of chronic degenerative diseases such as hypertension, obesity and diabetes *mellitus* (MARTINS, 96). In obese individuals, there are frequent alterations in the action of certain enzymes and in lipid metabolism, such as hypertriglyceridemia, low plasma HDL-c concentrations and an increase in small, dense LDL-c particles (FISBERG et al., 2006).

From a metabolic point of view, triglycerides stored in adipose tissue are the body's largest energy source, surpassing glycogen, due to their more compact structure, higher energy density and hydrophobic nature (SANTOS et al., 2006).

Hypertriglyceridemia is caused by increased synthesis of apolipoprotein C-III, which interferes with the action of LPL. This enzyme is synthesized in various tissues, mainly in adipose tissue and striated muscle. LPL hydrolyzes the triglycerides in the VLDL-c particle and chylomicrons, releasing fatty acids that can be taken up by adipocytes.

In addition, apolipoprotein C-III interferes with the uptake of VLDL-c remnants by LDL-c receptors in liver cells, leading to the accumulation of triglycerides in the bloodstream (SANTOS et al., 2006).

Insulin and cortisol are the main hormones regulating LPL activity. Insulin stimulates LPL activity in adipose tissue under anabolic conditions, while in striated and cardiac muscle, activity remains high or increases under catabolc conditions. Cortisol acts synergistically with insulin in the induction of LPL in adipose tissue. On the other hand, LPL is inhibited by testosterone, catecholamines and tumor necrosis factor (LOPEZ et al., 2005).

One of the mechanisms suggesting a reduction in plasma HDL-c levels ir hypertriglycemic states is that the triglyceride-enriched particles of HDL may be more unstable in the circulation because their apoproteins are more loosely adhered especially apo A-I, or due to dysfunctional LPL, with reduced activity, which can reduce the availability of the surface constituents of triglyceride-enriched lipoproteins, necessary for the formation of nascent HDL particles (CASELLA, 2007).

The need for HDL-c values above 50 mg/dl is due to the protective effect of this particle, through antioxidant enzymes that can prevent an initial inflammatory process. The increase in LDL-c due to a higher intake of saturated fatty acids and cholesterol by obese individuals leads to suppression of the activity of cell receptors for LDL, with its consequent accumulation in the circulation (FERREIRA, 2006). The metabolic alterations involved in MS are responsible for the higher incidence of smaller and denser LDL particles, establishing a strong link between this type of lipoprotein and endothelial dysfunction and consequent atherosclerotic disease (CASELLA, 2007).

In reverse cholesterol transport, most of the production of apo ipoprotein A-I, the fundamental constituent of nascent HDL particles, comes from the liver. LPL acts on VLDL and QM, detaching surface components of these lipoproteins, such as free cholesterol, phospholipids and apolipoproteins, giving rise to pre-beta HDL, or dissociated apolipoproteins A-1, which are responsible for the removal of excess cholesterol from peripheral cells through cell membranes. This remission occurs thanks to interaction with the membrane receptors ABC A-1 (ATP *biding cassette transporter* A-1) and SR-BI (CASELLA, 2007).

Once cholesterol has been captured, it is esterified by the enzyme lecithin-cholesterol acyltransferase (LCAT), located on the surface of HDL, and converted into cholesteryl ester, which fills the interior of the particle, leaving it with a spheroical shape, giving rise to HDL-3. The process is continued by the cholesterol ester transfer protein (CETP) (WAJCHENBERG, 2000), which captures triglycerides from the lipoproteins that contain QM, VLDL and LDL, transforming the HDL into even larger, globular HDL, known as HDL-2. CETP is responsible for the exchange of cholesteryl ester for triglycerides between HDL and VLDL/LDL. Triglyceride-rich HDL-2s are metabolized by hepatic LPL, which favours the subsequent repopulation of esterified cholesterol from their nucleus by SR-BI receptors. The remaining HDL components return to the interstitium, restarting the cholesterol removal cycle. The cholesterol from the periphery, now in the liver, is eliminated by the bile (CASELLA, 2007).

Studies suggest that a probable mechanism of atherosclerosis is the association of diabetes *mellitus* with factors such as dyslipidemia, insulin resistance and the direct toxic effects of glucose on the arteries (BAHIA et al., 2006).

Adhesion is achieved through cell surface proteins that are expressed in small quantities by endothelial cells and in the presence of inflammatory cytokines this response is increased. After adhesion, transmigration to the arterial intima occurs, accentuating the inflammatory response. Macrophages express receptors for modified lipoproteins (GOTTLIEB, 2005), engulfing minimally oxidized LDL particles, forming foam cells. These oxidized LDL molecules stimulate the production of pro-inflammatory molecules by endothelial cells, including leukocyte adhesion molecules and macrophage colony-stimulating factor (M-CSF), and inhibit the production of NO (BAHIA et al., 2006). T lymphocytes produce inflammatory cytokines, such as interferon gamma and tumor necrosis factor beta (TNF-в), which stimulate macrophages, endothelial cells and smooth muscle cells (GOTTLIEB, 2005).

If the inflammatory process persists, more leukocytes enter, activating the T lymphocytes, giving rise to a dense extracellular matrix which is a characteristic lesion of advanced atherosclerosis. This process that generates atherosclerosis can also rupture this atheroma plaque, causing acute thrombotic complications, through the proteolytic action of macrophages, which degrade collagen, responsible for the resistance of the fibrous layer that protects the plaque, leaving it susceptible to rupture (BAHIA et al., 2006).

Drug Treatment for Dyslipidemia

The dyslipidemia present in MS has low HDL-c levels, high triglyceride levels and, in some cases, altered LDL-c levels.
Statins

HMG-CoA reductase inhibitors are a notable class of cholesterol-lowering drugs and have been associated with a significant reduction in cardiovascular morbidity and mortality for patients undergoing primary or secondary prevention of coronary heart disease (FONSECA, 2005).

They are the first-choice drugs for the treatment of MS dyslipidemia, and their mechanism of action is based on the inhibition of HMG-CoA reductase and the blocking of triglyceride synthesis in the liver (I DIRETRIZ BRASILEIRA, 2005).

Most of the statins used today are metabolized in the liver via cytochrome P450 and most of the drugs used in cardiology and clinical medicine are metabolized via this route and when they are used simultaneously they can interfere with serum statin levels (BORGES, 2005).

The efficacy of statins is demonstrated by their ability to reduce cardiovascular morbidity and mortality and lower LDL cholesterol levels. There is an improvement in endothelial function by increasing the bioavailability of NO, increasing the activity of eNOS, anti-inflammatory effects, with a decrease in the expression of adhesion molecules and anti-oxidants (WASSMAN, 2004).

Nicotinic acid in combination with statins at lower doses is very effective in raising HDL-C, reducing LDL-C, triglycerides and small, dense LDL. It can also be considered much safer than the combination of statin and fibrate (BORGES, 2005).

One of the adverse effects of statins is rhabdomyolysis, with muscle toxicity. There are several reasons for this effect, such as: statins cause depletion of intermediate metabolites of cholesterol synthesis; they induce cell apoptosis and can cause alterations in chloride conductance channels within myocytes (ROSENDO et al., 2007).

Fibrates

They are PPAR-a agonists, modulate the genes that increase the expression of lipoprotein lipase, apolipoprotein AI and AII and reduce apolipoprotein CII, thus reducing triglycerides and increasing HDL-c (I DIRETRIZ BRASILEIRA, 2005).

Hypoglycemic drugs generally affect different classes of lipoproteins, making it difficult to say whether raising HDL alone would reduce cardiovascular risk (SANTOS, 2001).

In a clinical trial of secondary prevention in men with isolated HDL-cholesterol reduction, in which genfibrozil was used, LDL levels remained unchanged, HDL-cholesterol levels increased by 6% and triglyceride levels were reduced by 31%. In the multivariate analysis, HDL level during treatment was the only variable significantly associated with risk reduction, but it only explained 23% of the benefit obtained. This finding suggests that the effects of fibrate are not related to changes in lipid levels, so it cannot be said that other drugs developed to increase HDL levels would bring the same benefit (POZZAN et al., 2004).

They are drugs of first choice for patients with only high triglyceride levels (ARANCETA et al., 2003).

Nicotinic Acid

Drug intervention aimed at raising HDL levels is not yet recommended, given the lack of conclusive scientific evidence and the shortage of suitable drugs. To date, nicotinic acid is the drug with the greatest power to raise HDL levels, although it is associated with limiting side effects (POZZAN et al., 2004).

It acts by reducing LDL-c triglyceride levels and increasing HDL-c. Side effects may include heat and facial flushing (I DIRETRIZ BRASILEIRA, 2005).

Non-drug treatment of Metabolic Syndrome (MS)

The adoption of a diet plan to reduce weight, combined with physical exercise, are considered first choice therapies for the treatment of patients with metabolic syndrome, with the expectation of reducing abdominal circumference and visceral fat, improving insulin sensitivity, lowering plasma glucose levels and even delaying the onset of diabetes. A reduction in blood pressure and triglyceride levels is also expected, with an increase in HDL-c (I DIRETRIZ BRASILEIRA, 2005). These conservative, non-pharmacological treatments, such as diet therapy and physical exercise, reduce visceral obesity and insulin resistance with various benefits for the clinical manifestations of MS, such as improved lipid profile, glycemic control, blood pressure, among others (GELONEZE et al., 2006).

The primary objective of nutritional therapy is to limit the intake of saturated fats, as they are the main determining factor in the increase in p asma LDL-c concentrations, as they inhibit plasma clearance and are associated with altered insulin action, increased secretion of inflammatory cytokines, with a risk of impaired glucose tolerance and an increase in fasting glucose levels of this lipoprotein, as well as allowing more cholesterol to enter these particles. The lipids that contribute most tc this increase are trans fatty acid isomers, which are produced during the hydrogenation process of vegetable oils. They can increase the risk of cardiovascular disease and diabetes *mellitus* by modifying the lipid profile, decreasing HDL-c concentrations and increasing those of LDL-c and lipoprotein (a) (SANTOS et al., 2006).

Individuals with metabolic syndrome must adopt a healthy eating plan and have their metabolic profile determined in order to obtain effective nutritional therapy. In high quantities, omega-6 fatty acids can cause small reductions in serum HDL-c and triglyceride concentrations, as well as being more susceptible to oxidation. Omega-3 can lower triglyceride concentrations by reducing the synthesis of VLD_-c, as well as decreasing platelet adhesiveness and promoting a small reduction in blood pressure. Monounsaturated fats strengthen LDL-c particles, making them less prone to oxidation. Insulin sensitivity is improved with diets rich in monounsaturated or polyunsaturated fats, compared to those rich in saturated fats (SANTOS et al., 2006).

Diets rich in carbohydrates are associated with increased plasma concentrations of triglycerides and PAI-1, as well as a reduction in HDL-c, lower fibrinolysis and decreased sensitivity to insulin. Diets rich in fiber are associated with a lower risk of cardiovascular disease and type 2 diabetes *mellitus*. In addition, dietary fiber improves glycemic response and prandial insulin concentrations. One of the mechanisms by which soluble fibers improve cardiovascular risk is by slowing down intestinal transit and reducing cholesterol absorption. Insoluble fibers increase satiety, helping to reduce energy intake and may reduce body weight (SANTOS et al., 2006).

Replacing animal protein with soy protein lowers blood concentrations of total cholesterol and LDL-c in hypercholesterolemic individuals. Individuals with MS should limit salt intake, which can impair insulin sensitivity, raise blood pressure and increase calciuria. Calcium, potassium and magnesium seem to reduce the risk of systemic arterial hypertension, coronary artery disease and type 2 diabetes *mellitus* (BARRETO, 2005).

Low magnesium concentrations are associated with decreased insulin sensitivity, metabolic syndrome and type 2 diabetes *mellitus*. Foods rich in potassium and low in sodium can be recommended for hypertensive patients. Potassium can exert antihypertensive effects, have a protective action against cardiovascular damage, and serve as an auxiliary measure in patients undergoing diuretic therapy. Potassium chloride supplements can be used in patients with salt restriction, but should be used with caution in patients susceptible to hyperpotassemia, taking angiotensin-converting enzyme inhibitors (ACEIs), or angiotensin II receptor blockers (KOHLMANN, 1999).

Chronic exposure to glucose and free fatty acids can inhibit insulin secretion. According to El-Assaad's research group, type 2 diabetics have fewer cells due to greater stimulation of apoptosis, which can be induced by high concentrations of free fatty acids and glucose (SANTOS et al., 2006).

The diet of diabetics should be individualized according to their daily caloric needs, physical activity and eating habits. This alone would reduce three of the risk factors for cardiovascular disease, such as obesity, dyslipidemia, which is present in around a third of diabetics, and hypertension. A low-calorie diet improves insulin sensitivity and reduces hyperglycemia, regardless of weight loss (BATISTA, 2006).

Chronic physical exercise improves insulin sensitivity in healthy individuals, obese non-diabetics and type 1 and 2 diabetics (CIOLAC, 2004), reduces hyperinsulinemia, increases muscle glucose uptake, improves lipid profile and hypertension, as well as the resulting feeling of physical and psychological well-being; it can also contribute to weight loss. Reports in the literature suggest that physical exercise induces a decrease in triglyceride levels of 11 to 16%, in cholesterol of 3 to 10% and an increase in HDL-cholesterol of 3% (ARAUJO et al., 2000).

During exercise, the need for greater energy consumption, which will stimulate and capture glucose, improving and sensitizing insulin, also causes the oxidation of fatty acids in the circulation, providing ATP for the muscles during and after the activity. The effect of physical activity on insulin sensitivity has been shown to last between 12 and 48 hours, after which it can return to its initial levels in three to five days without exercise, requiring regular physical activity (PAULI et al., 2006).

Modification of inadequate eating behavior and weight loss, associated with regular physical activity, are considered first-choice therapies for the treatment of metabolic syndrome (MCLELLAN et al., 2006). The start of drug treatment is indicated when diet and increased physical activity are unable to normalize fasting and postprandial blood glucose values and glycosylated hemoglobin (ARAUJO et al., 2000).

The main objective of dietary changes in the approach to MS is to reduce the risk of diabetes and cardiovascular disease (SBEM, 2006).

3 FINAL CONSIDERATIONS

Metabolic syndrome is an important cardiovascular risk factor and the prevention of these complications must be based on the early identification of individuals at risk. The presence of MetS and its risk factors, especially insulin resistance, are related to the distribution of body fat, which is becoming increasingly prevalent in younger individuals, due to the lifestyle adopted by the current population, which is very sedentary.

In obese people, glucose tolerance may be reduced due to the antagonistic action of resistin on insulin. Because it is related to the amount of adipose tissue, leptin is increased in overweight people and also modulates insulin action and sensitivity. Hyperleptinemia may be a pathogenetic factor in MS.

The treatment of MS is based initially on lifestyle changes, such as adopting a diet plan to reduce weight and promoting increased physical activity.

The antihypertensive treatment best suited to MS patients is ACE inhibitors, due to their insulin-sensitizing action, with improvements in endothelial function. These drugs can be used as monotherapy or in association with diuretics, which are not recommended as monotherapy in MS due to the possibility of generating glucose intolerance, as well as beta-blockers. If there is a contraindication to the use of LECAs, one option is angiotensin receptor antagonists, which have great potential benefits.

Due to the reduction in cardiovascular morbidity and improvement in endothelial function, the first choice treatment for dyslipidemia in MS is statins.

The therapy for diabetes associated with MS is metformin, which can reduce LDL-c and increase HDL-c, improve endothelial function, reduce blood pressure and help with weight loss. The addition of insulin is indicated in cases of inadequate therapy and failure to achieve the expected goals.

4 REFERENCES

AMERICAN DIABETES ASSOCIATION. **Standards of medical care in diabetes**. Diabetes care: v. 28,.p.4-59, 510-36., 2005.

ANDRADE, B. M. C; MENDES, C. M. C.; ARAUJO, L. M. B. Floating weight in the treatment of obese women. **Arq Bras Endocrinol Metab.** , v.48,n. 2, p.276-281 2004.

APPOLINARIO, J. C; BACALTCHUK, J. Pharmacological treatment of eating disorders. **Rev bras psiquiatr.**, v. 24, suppl. 3, p. 54-59, 2002.

ARANCETA, J.; FOZ, G.; MANTILLA, J.; MONEREO, M. Consensus document: obesity and cardiovascular risk. **Clin Investa Arterioscl.**, v. 15, n. 5, p. 196-233, 2003

ARAUJO, L. M. B.; BRITTO, M. M. S.; PORTO DA CRUZ, T. R. Treatment of type 2 diabetes mellitus: new options. **Arq Bras Endocrinol Metabol.**, v. 44, n 6, 509-518 2000.

ARPA GAMEZ, A.; GONZALEZ SOTOLONGO, O.; ROLDOS CUZA, E.. Metabolic syndrome as a risk factor for endothelial dysfunction. **Rev Cub Med Mil.**, v. 36, n. 1, 2007.

ATALA, S. Insulin resistance and metabolic syndrome in type 1 diabetes mellitus. **Arq Bras Endocrinol Metab.**, v. 50, n. 2, p. 250-263, 2006.

ATTUX, C.; QUINTANA, M. I.; CHAVES, A. C. Weight gain, dyslipidemia and altered parameters for metabolic syndrome in patients with a first psychotic episode after a six-month follow-up. **Rev Bras Psiquiatr.**, v. 29, n. 4, p. 346349 2007.

BAHIA, L.; AGUIAR, L. G.; VILLELA, N.; BOTTINO, D.; GODOY-MATOS, A. F.; BOUSKELA. E. Effects of rosiglitasone on endothelial function in non-diabetic individuals with metabolic syndrome. **Arq Brasi Cardiol.**, v. 86, n. 5, p. 366-373 2006.

BARRETO, S. M., PINHEIRO, A. R. O., SICHIERI, R. Analysis of the World Health Organization's global strategy for food, physical activity and health. **Epidemiologia Servigo de Saude**, v.14, n.1 p.41-68. 2005.

BATISTA, M.; SILVIA P.; ROSADO, L.; TINOCO, A.; FRANCESCHINI, S. Dietary assessment of the patients detected with hyperglycemia in the Detection of Diabetes in Suspect Cases Campaign in Vigosa, MG. **Arq Bras Endocrinol Metabol**. Sao Paulo: v. 50, n. 6, p. 1041-1049, 2006.

BORGES, J. L. Combination of drugs: statins and niacin. **Arquivos Brasileiros de Cardiologia**. v. 85, suppl. 5, p. 36-41,2005.

BRASILEIRO-FILHO, G. **BOGLIOLO: PATHOLOGIA**. 8ª Ed. Rio de Janeiro: GUANABARA KOOGAN, 2011, 1524p.

BRUNTON, L. L.; LAZO, J. S.; PARKER, K.. Goodman & Gilman **The Pharmacological Basis of Therapeutics**. 12th Ed. Rio de Janeiro. McGraw-Hill, 2012, 2112p.

BURROWS A, R., LEIVA B, L., WEISTAUB, G. Metabolic syndrome in children and adolescents: association with insulin sensitivity and the magnitude and distribution of obesity. Rev. Med. Chile, v.135, n. 2, p.174-181, 2007.

CASTRO, S. H.; MATO, H. J. GOMES, M. B. Anthropometric parameters and metabolic syndrome in type 2 diabetes. **Arq bras, Endocrinol Metab.**, v. 50, n. 3, p. 450-455, 2006.

CIOLAC, E. G.; GUIMARAES, G. V. Physical exercise and metabolic syndrome: . Rev Bras Med Esporte , v.10, n.4, p. 319-324, 2004.

COUTINHO, W. Etiology of Obesity. ABESO (Brazilian Association for the Study of Obesity and Metabolic Syndromes), **ABESO Magazine**. 30. ed. 2007: Available at: <http://www.abeso.org.br/revista/revista30/etiologia_obesidade.htm> Accessed on: May 28, 2014.

CRISPIM, C. A.; ZALCMAN, I.; DATTILO, M.; PADILHA, G. H.; TUFIK, S.; MELLO, M T. Relationship between sleep and obesity: a literature review. **Arq Bras Endocrinol Metab.**, v.51, n.7, p. 1041-1049, 2007

I Diretriz Brasileira de Diagnostico e Tratamento da Sindrome Metabolica. **Arq Bras Cardiol.** v. 84, Suplemento I, 2005 . Available at: <http://www.sielo.br/scielo.php>. Accessed on: May 09, 2014.

DUARTE, A. C. G.; FAILLACE, G. B.; WADI, M. T.; PINHEIRO, R. **Sindrome metabolica: semiologia, bioquimica e prescrigao nutricional**. Rio de Janeiro: Axcel, p.255, 2005

EMEA, European Agency for the Evaluation of Medicinal Products. **Fourth General Activity Report of the European Agency for the Evaluation of Medicinal Products**. London, 1998. Available at: < http://www.emea.europa.eu/pdfs/general/direct/emeaar/ar98pt.pdf> Accessed on: June 10, 2014.

FARIA, A. N; FILHO, F. R; LERARIO, D. D; KOHLMANN, N.; FERREIRA, S. R; ZANELLA, M. T. Effects of Sibutramine on the Treatment of Obesity in Patients with Arterial Hypertension. **Arq. Bras. Cardiol.**, v.78, n.2, p. 176-180, 2002.

Treatment of Diabetes and Hypertension in Obese Patients. **Arq Bras Endocrinol Metab.**, v.46, n.2, p. 127-136. 2002.

FERREIRA, A P.I; FRANQA, N. M. Metabolic syndrome and cardiovascular risk factors in pre-pubertal children of different nutritional classifications and levels of insulin resistance. 142 f, 2006. **Dissertation (Master's Degree) - Universidade Catolica de Brasilia, 2006.**

FISBERG, M.; LEITE, C. C.; HERSZKOWICZ, N.; BARBATO, A.; COSTA, A. P. A. Obesity and metabolic syndrome in childhood and adolescence. Sao Paulo: **Federal University of Sao Paulo, 2006**. Available at: <http://br.monografias.com/trabalhos2/obesidade-sindrome-metabolica/obesidade-sindrome- metabolica.shtml>. Accessed on: May 28, 2008.

FONSECA, F. A. Helfenstein Pharmacokinetics of statins. **Arq. Bras. Cardiol.**, v.85, suppl.5, p. 9-14, 2005.

GALVAO, R.; KOHLMANN, O. J. Arterial hypertension in obese patients. **Rev Bras Hipertens**, v. 9, n. 3, p. 262-7, 2002.

GIGEK, G. O. Analysis of the lipoprotein lipase (LPL) Ser447Ter polymorphism and its association with history of morbidity and serum triglyceride levels in an elderly population in Sao Paulo. **XIII Congress of Scientific Initiation of UNIFESP - 2005. Molecular Basic Sciences 4. Sao Paulo,** 2005.

GUIMARAES, C.; PEREIRA, L. R; JUNIOR, N.; CESARINO, E. J.; ALMEIDA, C.; CARVALHO, D. QUEIROZ, R.. Tolerability and efficacy of fluoxetine, metformin and sibutramine in reducing anthropometric and metabolic parameters in obese patients. **Arq Bras Endocrinol.**, v.50.,n.6, p. 1020 2006.

GODOY-MATOS, A. F. The endocannabinoid system: a new paradigm n the metabolic syndrome treatment. **Arq Bras Endocrinol Metab.**, v.50, n.2, p. 390- 399, 2006.

GONZALEZ, O. S; ARPA, A. G. Sistema de pesquisa clinico Del sindrome metabolica. Rev Cub Med Mil., v.35, n. 3, p. 0-0, 2006.

GOTTLIEB, M. G.V.; BONARDI, G.; MORIGUCHI, E. H. Physiopathology and inflammatory aspects of atherosclerosis. **Scientia Medica. Porto Alegre**, v. 15, n. 3,p. 203207, 2005.

HALPERN, Alfredo. Evaluation of the efficacy, safety and tolerability of sibutramine in obese patients - a randomized double-blind study. **Rev. Hosp. Clin.** [online], v.57, n 3, pp. 98-102, 2002.

GARRIDO JUNIOR, A. B. Clinical experience with the combined use of sibutramine and orlistat in obese patients. **Arq Bras Endocrinol Metabol**, v.44, n. 1, p. 106-113, 2000.

HEIMANN, A. S. **The angiotensin I-converting enzyme gene influences changes in diabetes**. Sao Paulo, PhD Thesis, Faculty of Medicine, University of Sao Paulo. 2003.

KNOWLER, W.; CONNOR, B.; HAMMAN, R.; LACHIN, M.; WALKER, E.; NATHAN, D. Reduction in the incidence of type 2 diabetes with lifestyle intervent on or metformin. Diabetes Prevention Program Research Group. **N Engl J Med,** v. 346, n. 6, p. 393-403, 2006.

KOHLMANN JR., O. III Brazilian Consensus on Arterial Hypertension. **Arq Bras Endocrinol Metab.**, vol.43, n.4, pp. 247-249, 1999.

LAMOUNIER, R.. Endocannabinoid System: a New Understanding of Obesity and Related Disorders. **Brazilian Diabetes Society. 2006**. Available at: < http://www.diabetes.org.br/colunistas/dr-rodrigo-lamounier/sistema- endocannabincid-system-a-new-understanding-of-obesity-and-related-disorders>. Accessed on: June 25, 2014.

LOMBO, B.; SATIZABAL, C. L.; VILLALOBOS, C.; TIQUE, C.; WILLIAM, K. Prevalence of the metabolic syndrome in diabetic patients. **Acta Medica Colombiana [online],** v. 32, n. 1 p. 9-15, 2005. Available at: < http://www.scielo.org.co/pdf/amc/v32n1/v32n1a3.pdf>. Accessed on: May 12, 2014.

LOPEZ, P. J.; PRADILLA, L. P.; BRACHO, Yalil. The role of adipocytes in metabolic syndrome inflammation. **Acta Med Colomb.,** v. 30, n. 3, p. 137 - 140, 2005.

LOPEZ DE FEZ, C.M.; GAZTELU, M.T; BUBIO, T; CASTANO, A. Mecanismo de hipertension em obesidade. **Anales Sis San Navarra,** v.27, n.2, p. 211-219. 2004.

LOTTENBERG, S. A.; GLEZER, A.; TURATTI, L. A. Metabolic syndrome: identifying risk factors. **J. Pediatr.,** v.83, n.5, suppl., p. S204-S208 2007.

MACHADO, R. C. Cardiovascular risk in metabolic syndrome: estimation by different scores. **Rev Bras Clin Med**, v. 8, n. 3, p. 198-204, 2006.

MANCINI, M. C; HALPERN, A.. Pharmacological treatment of obesity. **Arq Bras Endocrinol Metab.**, v. 50, , n.5, p. 497-512, 2006.

MARTIN, M.; DIAZ, M; BAYO, M. Metformin in the treatment of type 2 diabetes with overweight or obesity. **An. Med. Interna (Madrid)**, v.22, n.12, p. 579-585. 2005..

MATOS, A. F. G.; MOREIRA, R. O; GUEDES, E. P. Neuroendocrinology of the metabolic syndrome. **Arq Bras Endocrinol Metab.,** v.47, n.4, p. 410-420, 2003.

MCLELLAN, K. C. Portero et al. Type 2 diabetes mellitus, metabolic syndrome and lifestyle modification: **Rev Nutr.** v.20, , n.5, p. 515-524, 2007.

MENDIVIL, C. O.. Orlistat and sibutramine in the management of metabolic syndrome. **Acta Med Colomb**, v. 30, n. 3, p. 168-170, 2005.

MION D JR, GOMES M A, F. N; IV Diretrizes Brasileiras de Hipertensao Arterial. **Arq Bras Cardiol**. v. 82, n. 4, p. 1-14, 2004.

MOLINA, M. C.; CUNHA R S, HERKENHOFF LF, MILL JG. Hypertension and salt intake in an urban population. **Rev Saude Publica**, v. 37, p.743-750, 2003.

MOREIRA, D. A. R. Metabolic Syndromes and Cardiac Arrhythmias: Obesity, Inflammation and Cardiac Arrhythmias. Sao Paulo: **Itajuba Medical School**, 2007.

NEUTEL, J. Effect of the renin-angiotensin system on thevessel wall: using ACE inhibition to improve endothelial function. **Journal of Human Hypertension,** v. 18, p.599-606, 2004.

PAGOTTO UBERTO, M.; GIOVANNI, C. D.; LUTZ BEAT, PASQUALI. R.. The emerging Role of the Endocannabinoid System in Endocrine Regulation and Energy Balance. **Endocrine Reviews,** .v. 27, n. 1, p. 73-100, 2006. Available at <http://edrv.endojournals.org/cgi/content/full/27/1/73> Accessed on: May 23, 2014

PAULI, J. R., SOUZA, L., ROGATTO, G. Glucocorticoids and metabolic syndrome: favorable aspects of physical exercise in this pathophysiology. **Rev. Port. Cien.**

Desp., v.6, n. 2, p.217-228, 2006.

PELLIZZARO, M. C; PANCHENIAK, E. F. R. Pharmaceutical assistance in the treatment of cardiovascular diseases and hypertension. **Infarma**, v. 15, r. 9-10, p. 2003, 2003

PESSUTO, J.; CARVALHO, E. C. Risk factors in individuals with hypertension: **Ver. Latino-Am. Enfermagem,** v.6, n. 1, p. 33-39, 1998.

PICON, P. X.; ZANATTA, C. M.; GERCHMAN, F.; ZELMANOVITZ, T.; GROSS, J. L.; CANANI, L. H. Analysis of the criteria for defining metabolic syndrome in patients with type 2 diabetes mellitus: **Arquivos Brasileiros de Endocrinologia e Metabologia,** v.50, n. 2, p. 264-270, 2006.

PIMENTA, E.; PASSARELLI, O.; BORELLI, F.; SOUSA, C. G; AMATO, V.; AMODEO, C.; PIEGAS, L. S. Metabolic syndrome in patients undergoing coronary artery bypass grafting: prevalence and marker of morbidity and mortality in the in-hospital period and after 30 days. **Arq. Bras. Cardiol.**, v.88, n. 4, p. 413-417, 2007.

PIVATTO, I.; BUSTOS, P.; AMIGO, H.; ACOSTA, A. M.; ARTEAGA, A. Association between proinsulin, insulin, proinsulin/insulin factor and insulin resistance index with metabolic syndrome. **Arquivos Brasileiros de Endocrinologia e Metabologia,** vol.51, n.7, p. 1128-1133, 2007.

PORTO, L. C. Role of orotic acid in cardiac energy metabolism in rats. Belo Horizonte,,xiv, 82p., 2007.p.**Thesis (Doctorate) - Federal University of Minas Gerais. Institute of Biological Sciences**. Postgraduate Program in Biological Sciences - Physiology and Pharmacology.

RANG, H. P.; DALE, M. M.;RITTER, J. M.; FLOWER, R. J.; HENDERSON, G. **Pharmacology.** 7ª Ed. Rio de Janeiro. Elsevier, 2011,441p.

REAVEN, GM; THE METABOLIC SYNDROME: IS THIS DIAGNOSIS NECESSARY?, **Am J Clin Nutr**, v. 83, n. 6, p. 1237-1247, 2006.

REGIDOR, E., GUTIERREZ, J.; BANEGAS, J. R; DOMINGUEZ, V.; RODRIGUEZ, F. Lifelong influence of socioeconomic circumstances, physical inactivity and obesity on the presence of metabolic syndrome: **Revista Espanhola Salud Publica**, v.81, n.1, p. 25-31, 2007.

RIBEIRO FILHO, F.; MARIOSA, L. S; FERREIRA, S.; ZANELLA, M. T. Visceral fat and metabolic syndrome: more than a simple association. **Arquivos Brasileiros de Endocrinologia e Metabologia**. 2.ed. Sao Paulo, v.50, p. 230-238, 2006.

ROSENDO, A. B.; DAL-PIZZOL, F.; FIEGENBAUM, M.; ALMEIDA, S. Pharmacogenetics and anti-inflammatory effect of HMG-CoA reductase inhibitors. **Arq Bras Endocrinol Metab.,**. v.51, n.4, p. 520-525, 2007.

SALAROLI, L. B.; BARBOSA, G. C; MILL, J. G; MOLINA, M. C. Prevalence of metabolic syndrome in a population-based study, Vitoria, ES - Brazil. **Arquivos Brasileiros de Endocrinologia e Metabologia**, v.51, n.7, p. 1143-1152, 2007.

SALAZAR, D. I. M. Anti-hypertensive drugs in metabolic syndrome. **Acta Medica Colombiana**, v. 30, n.3, p. 170-173, 2005.

SANTOMAURO, A. C.; UGOLINI, M. R; SANTOMAURO, A. T.; SOUTO, R. P. Metformin and AMPK: an old drug and a new enzyme in the context of metabolic syndrome. **Arq Bras Endocrinol e Metab.**, v. 52,n. 1, p. 120-125, 2008.

SANTOS, C. R. B.; PORTELLA, E. S; AVILA, S. S; SOARES, E. Dietary factors in the prevention and treatment of comorbidities associated with metabolic syndrome. **Rev.Nutr.**, v.19, n.3, p. 389-401,2006.

SANTOS, R. D. III Diretrizes Brasileiras Sobre Dislipidemias e Diretriz de Prevengao da Aterosclerose do Departamento de Aterosclerose da Sociedade Brasileira de Cardiologia. **Arq Bras Cardiol**, v.77, suppl.3, p. 1-48. 2001.

SCHAAN, B. D. Role of protein kinase C in the development of vascular complications of diabetes mellitus. **Arq Bras Endocrinol Metab.**, vol.47, n. 6, p. 654662, 2003.

VALDELAMAR, L.; RODRIGUEZ, M.; BERMUDEZ, V.. Pharmacological treatment of obesity: present, past and future. **AVFT**, v.26, n.1, p.10-20, 2007.

WAJCHENBERG, B. L. Adipose tissue as an endocrine gland. **Arquivos Brasileiros de Endocrinologia e Metabologia**, v.44, n.1, p. 13-20, 2000.

WASSERMAN, L., All of statistics: a concise course in statistical inference, **Springer**, New York, 2004.

WEARLEY, R. Meabolic syndrome. Device or devisise? **Cardiac care**. 2007. Available at: <http://www.acc.org/membership/cca/pdfs/newsletter_july07.pdf> Accessed on: May 08, 2014.

ZOU, M.H; KIRKPATRICK, S; DAVIS, B; NELSON, J; WILES, W; SCHALATTNER, **U.** Activation of the AMP-activated protein kinase by the anti-diabetic drug metformin in vivo - role of mitochondrial reactive nitrogen species. **J. Biol. Chem**. p.279, 2004.

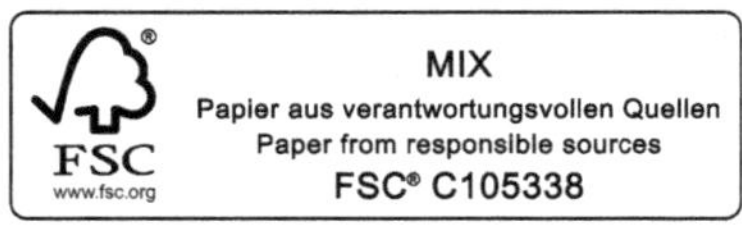

Printed by Books on Demand GmbH, Norderstedt / Germany